The Ultimate KETO Chaffle Cooking Guide

Delicious Chaffle Recipes For Everyone

Lily Sherman

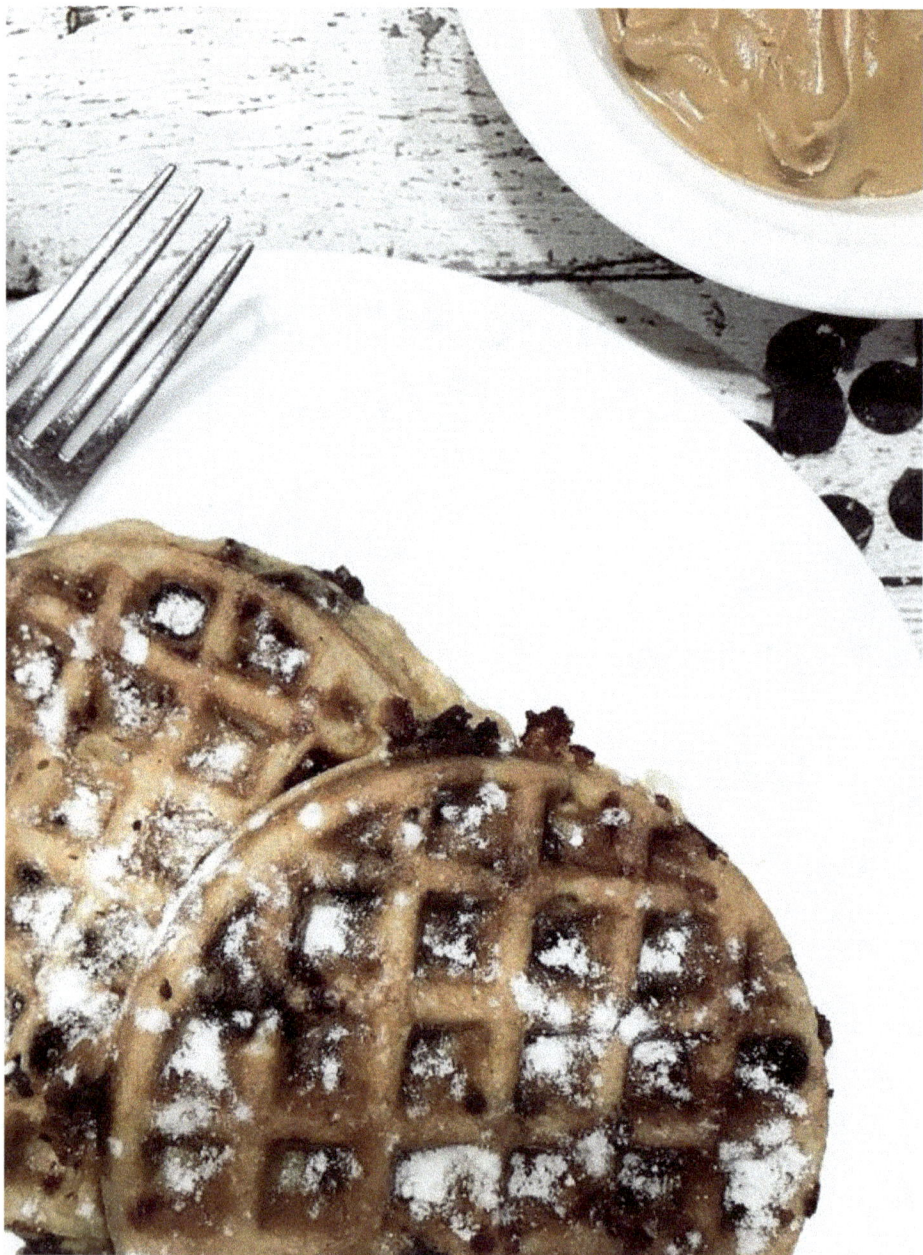

Table of contents

Layered Cheese Chaffles

Cooking: 5 Minutes

Servings: 1

Ingredients

- 1 organic egg, beaten
- 1/3 cup of Cheddar cheese, shredded
- ½ teaspn ground flaxseed
- ¼ teaspn organic baking powder
- 2 tbsps Parmesan cheese, shredded

Directions

1. Preheat now a mini waffle iron and then grease it.
2. Place all the ingredients except Parmesan and beat until well combined in a bowl.
3. Place half the Parmesan cheese in the bottom of Preheat waffle iron.
4. Place half of the egg mixture over cheese and top with the remaining Parmesan cheese.
5. Cook for about 3-minutes or until golden brown.
6. Serve warm.

Nutrition:

Calories: 264, Net Carb: 1, Fat: 20g, Saturated Fat: 11.1g, Carbohydrates: 2.1g, Dietary Fiber: 0.4g, Sugar: 0.6g, Protein: 18.9g

Egg-free Psyllium Husk Chaffles

Cooking: 4 Minutes

Servings: 1

Ingredients

- 1 ounce of Mozzarella cheese, shredded
- 1 tbspn cream cheese, softened
- 1 tbspn psyllium husk powder

Directions

1. Preheat now a waffle iron and then grease it.
2. Place all ingredients and pulse in a blender until a slightly crumbly mixture forms.
3. Place the mixture into Preheat nowed waffle iron and cook for about 4 minutes or until golden brown.
4. Serve warm.

Nutrition:

Calories: 137, Net Carb: 1.3gm Fat: 8.8gm Saturated Fat: 2gm
Carbohydrates: 1.3g, Dietary Fiber: 0g, Sugar: 0g, Protein: 9.5g

Mozzarella & Almond Flour Chaffles

Cooking: 8 Minutes

Servings: 2

Ingredients

- ½ cup Mozzarella cheese, shredded
- 1 large organic egg
- 2 tbsps blanched almond flour
- ¼ teaspn organic baking powder

Directions

1. Preheat now a mini waffle iron and then grease it.
2. In a bowl, place all ingredients and with a fork, Mix well until well combined.
3. Place half of the mixture into Preheat nowed waffle iron and cook for about 4 minutes or until golden brown.
4. Repeat now with the remaining mixture.
5. Serve warm.

Nutrition:

Calories: 98, Net Carb: 1.4g, Fat: 7.1g, Saturated Fat: 1g, Carbohydrates: 2.2g, Dietary Fiber: 0.8g, Sugar: 0.2g, Protein: 7g

Cheddar & Egg White Chaffles

Cooking: 12 Minutes

Servings: 4

Ingredients

- 2 egg whites
- 1 cup Cheddar cheese, shredded

Directions

1. Preheat now a mini waffle iron and then grease it.
2. Place the egg whites and cheese and stir to combine in a tiny bowl.
3. Place ¼ of the mixture into Preheat nowed waffle iron and cook for about 4 minutes or until golden brown.
4. Repeat now with the remaining mixture.
5. Serve warm.

Nutrition:

Calories: 122, Net Carb: 0.5g, Fat: 9.4g, Carbohydrates: 0.5g, Dietary Fiber: 0g Sugar: 0.3g, Protein: 8.8g

Basic Recipe For Cheese Chaffles

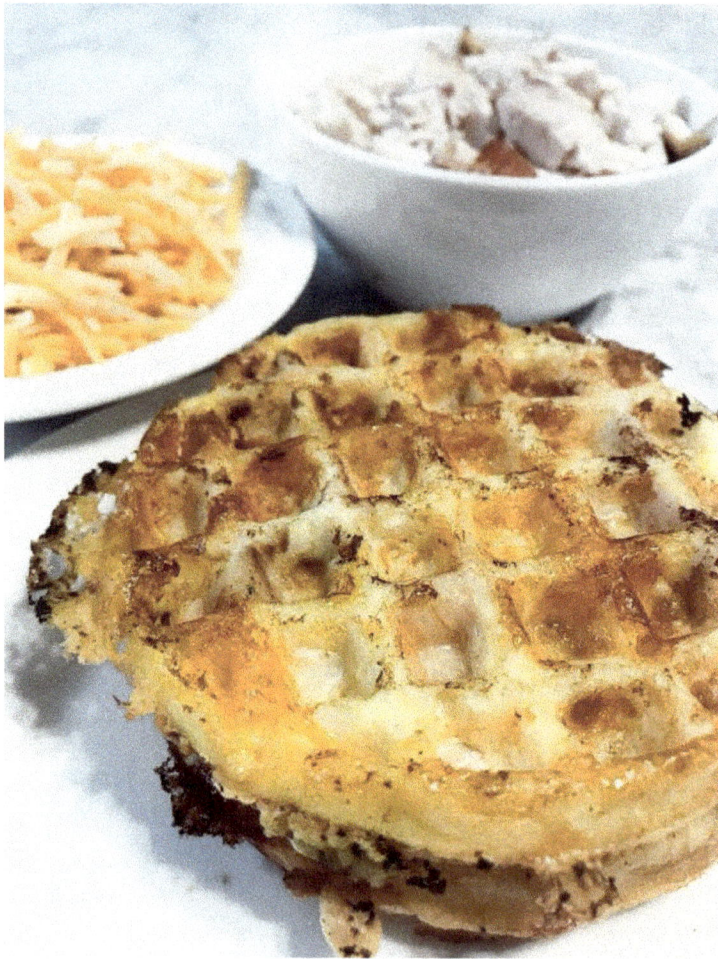

Cooking: 15 minutes

Servings: 2

Ingredients

- 1 medium or large egg
- 50 g of grated mozzarella (fresh, self-grated is less suitable) cheesebutter
- Salt
- Pepper

Directions

1. While the chaffle iron is heating, whisk the egg and fold in the fresh mozzarella.
2. Season with pepper and salt and add a little butter to the iron. As soon as it is Melt nowed and well distributed, add the dough and bake the cheese chaffles until they are golden brown and crispy.
3. Salty chaffles of this type taste both warm and cold.

Chocolate & Almond Chaffle

Cooking: 12 Minutes

Servings: 3

Ingredients

- 1 egg
- ¼ cup mozzarella cheese, shredded
- 1 oz. cream cheese
- 2 teaspns sweetener
- 1 teaspn vanilla
- 2 tbsps cocoa powder
- 1 teaspn baking powder
- 2 tbsps almonds, chopped
- 4 tbsps almond flour

Directions

1. Blend all the ingredients in a bowl while your waffle maker is Preheat nowing.
2. Pour some of the mixture into your waffle maker.
3. Close and cook for 4 minutes.
4. Transfer the chaffle to a plate. Let cool for 2 minutes.
5. Repeat steps using the remaining mixture.

Nutrition:

Calories 1, Total Fat 13.1g, Saturated Fat 5g, Cholesterol 99mg, Sodium 99mg, Potassium 481mg, Total Carbohydrate 9.1g, Dietary Fiber 3.8g, Protein 7.8g, Total Sugars 0.8g

Cheddar & Almond Flour Chaffles

Preparation: 10 minutes

Cooking: 10 Minutes

Servings: 2

Ingredients

- 1 large organic egg, beaten
- ½ cup Cheddar cheese, shredded
- 2 tbsps almond flour

Directions

1. Preheat now a mini waffle iron and then grease it.
2. Place the egg, Cheddar cheese, and almond flour and beat until well combined in a bowl.
3. Place half of the mixture into Preheat nowed waffle iron and cook for about 5 minutes or until golden brown.
4. Repeat now with the remaining mixture.
5. Serve warm.

Nutrition:

Calories 398, Total Fat 13.8 g, Saturated Fat 5.1 g, Cholesterol 200 mg, Total Carbs 3.6 g, Fiber 1 g, Sugar 1.3 g, Sodium 272 mg, Potassium 531 mg, Protein 51.8 g

Parmesan Garlic Chaffles

Preparation: 10 minutes

Cooking: 5 minutes

Servings: 1

Ingredients

- 1/2 cup shredded Mozzarella cheese
- 1 whole egg, beaten
- 1/4 cup grated Parmesan cheese
- 1 teaspn Italian Seasoning
- 1/4 teaspn garlic powder

Directions

1. Start pre-heating your waffle maker, and let's start preparing the batter.
2. Add in all the ingredients, except for the Mozzarella cheese to a bowl and whisk. Add in the cheese and Mix well until well combined.
3. Spray your waffle plates with nonstick spray and add half the batter to the center. Close the lid and cooking for 3-5 min, depending on how crispy you want your Chaffles.

4. Serve with a drizzle of olive oil, grated Parmesan cheese and fresh chopped parsley or basil.

Nutrition:

Net Carbs: 6g; Calories: 340; Total Fat: 20g; Saturated Fat: 4g; Protein: 32g; Carbs: 8g; Fiber: 2g; Sugar: 2g

Key Lime Chaffle

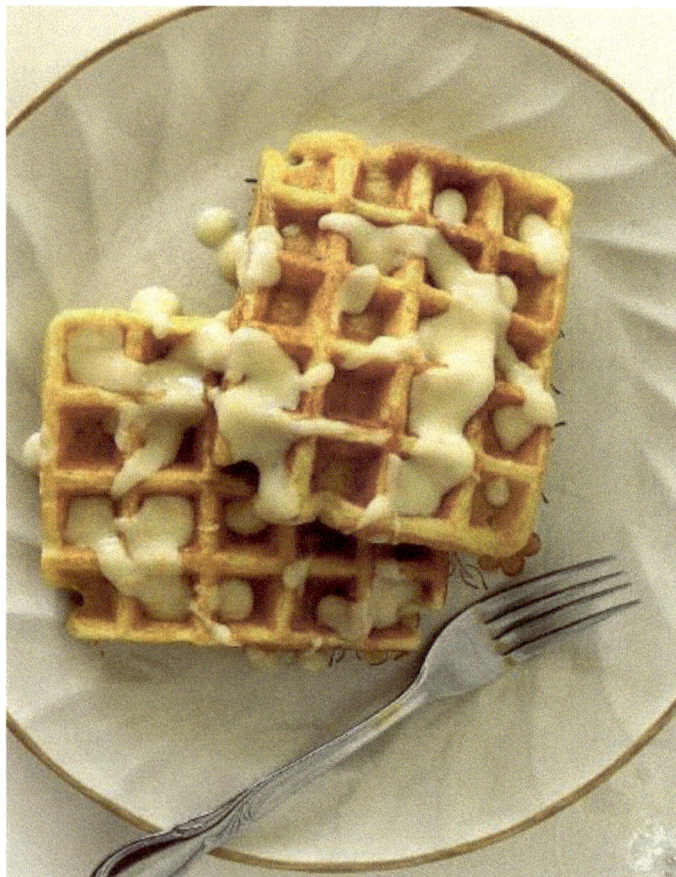

Preparation: 10 minutes

Cooking: 5 minutes

Servings: 2

Ingredients

Chaffle:

- 1 egg
- 2 tsp. cream cheese room temp
- 1 tsp. powdered sweetener swerve or monkfruit
- 1/2 tsp. baking powder
- 1/2 tsp. lime zest
- 1/4 cup Almond flour
- 1/2 tsp. lime extract or 1 tsp. fresh squeezed lime juice
- Pinch of salt

Cream Cheese Lime Frosting:

- 4 oz. cream cheese softened
- 4 tbs butter
- 2 tsp. powdered sweetener swerve or monkfruit
- 1 tsp. lime extract
- 1/2 tsp. lime zest

Directions

1. Preheat now the mini waffle iron.
2. In a blender add all the chaffle ingredients and blend on high until the mixture is smooth and creamy.

3. Cooking each chaffle about 3 to 4 minutes until it's golden brown.
4. While the chaffles are cooking, the frosting.
5. In a tiny bowl, combine all the frosting and mix ingredients until smooth.
6. Allow the chaffles to completely cool before frosting them.

Nutrition:

Net Carbs: 2.4g; Calories: 368.5; Total Fat: 26.6g; Saturated Fat: 10.1g; Protein: 19.5g; Carbs: 2.7g; Fiber: 0.3g; Sugar: 2g

Light & Crispy Chaffles

Preparation: 10 minutes

Cooking: 5 minutes

Servings: 2

Ingredients
- 1 egg
- 1/3 cup of cheddar
- 1/4 teaspn baking powder
- 1/2 teaspn ground flaxseed
- Shredded parmesan cheese on top and bottom.

Directions
1. Mix now the ingredients and cooking in a mini waffle iron for 4-5 minutes until crispy.
2. Once cool, enjoy your light and crisp Keto waffle.
3. You can experiment with seasonings to the initial mixture depending on your taste buds' mood.

Nutrition:

Net Carbs: 1.9g; Calories: 160.7; Total Fat: 8.2g; Saturated Fat: 8.1g; Protein: 19.3g; Carbs: 2.4g; Fiber: 0.5g; Sugar: 1.4g

Chaffle Sandwich With Bacon and Egg

Preparation: 10 minutes

Cooking: 5 minutes

Servings: 1

Ingredients

- 1 large egg
- 1/2 cup of shredded cheese
- thick-cut bacon
- fried egg
- sliced cheese

Directions

1. Preheat now your waffle maker.
2. In a tiny mixing bowl, mix egg and shredded cheese. Stir until well combined.
3. Pour one half of the waffle batter into your waffle maker. Cooking for 3-4 minutes or until golden brown. Repeat now with the second half of the batter.
4. In a large pan over medium heat, cooking the bacon until crispy.

5. In the same skillet, in 1 tbsp. of reserved bacon drippings, fry the egg over medium heat. Cooking until desired doneness.
6. Assemble the sandwich, and enjoy!

Nutrition:

Net Carbs: 5.7g; Calories: 358.8; Total Fat: 25.1g; Saturated Fat: 4.3g; Protein: 26g; Carbs: 7.2g; Fiber: 1.5g; Sugar: 3.6g

Garlic And Parsley Chaffles

Cooking: 5 Minutes

Servings: 1

Ingredients

- 1 large egg
- 1/4 cup cheese mozzarella
- 1 tsp. coconut flour
- ¼ tsp. baking powder
- ½ tsp. garlic powder
- 1 tbsp. minutesced parsley

For Serving:

- 1 Poach egg
- 4 oz. smoked salmon

Directions

1. Switch on your waffle maker and let it Preheat now.
2. Grease waffle maker with cooking spray.
3. Mix egg, mozzarella, coconut flour, baking powder, and garlic powder, parsley to a mixing bowl until combined well.

4. Pour batter in circle chaffle maker.
5. Close the lid.
6. Cook for about 2-3 minutes or until the chaffles are cooked.
7. Serve with smoked salmon and poached egg.
8. Enjoy!

Nutrition:

Protein: 45% 140 kcal, Fat: 51% 160 kcal, Carbohydrates: 4% 14 kcal

Cream Cheese Chaffle

Cooking: 8 Minutes

Servings: 2

Ingredients

- 1 egg, beaten
- 1 oz. cream cheese
- ½ teaspn vanilla
- 4 teaspns sweetener
- ¼ teaspn baking powder
- Cream cheese

Directions

1. Preheat now your waffle maker.
2. Add all the ingredients in a bowl.
3. Mix well.
4. Pour half of the batter into your waffle maker.
5. Seal the device.
6. Cook for 4 minutes.
7. Remove now the chaffle from your waffle maker.
8. Make the second one using the same steps.

9. Spread remaining cream cheese on top before serving.

Nutrition:

Calories 169, Total Fat 14.3g, Saturated Fat 7.6g, Cholesterol 195mg, Sodium 147mg, Potassium 222mg, Total Carbohydrate 4g, Dietary Fiber 4g, Protein 7.7g, Total Sugars 0.7g

Cereal and walnut Chaffle

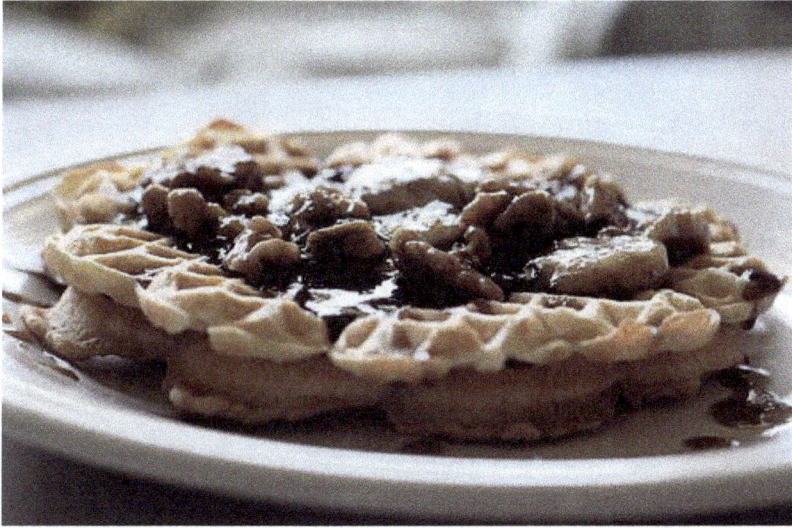

Preparation: 5 mins

Cooking: 6 mins

Servings: 2

Ingredients

- 1 milliliter of cereal flavoring
- ¼ tsp baking powder
- 1 tsp granulated swerve
- 1/8 tsp xanthan gum

33

- 1 tbsp butter (Melt nowed)
- ½ tsp coconut flour
- 2 tbsp toasted walnut (chopped)
- 1 tbsp cream cheese
- 2 tbsp almond flour
- 1 large egg (beaten)
- ¼ tsp cinnamon
- 1/8 tsp nutmeg

Directions

1. Plug your waffle maker to Preheat now it and spray it with a non-stick spray.
2. In a mixing bowl, whisk together the egg, cereal flavoring, cream cheese and butter.
3. In another mixing bowl, combine the coconut flour, almond flour, cinnamon, nutmeg, swerve, xanthan gum and baking powder.
4. Pour the egg mixture into the flour mixture and Mix well until you form a smooth batter.
5. Fold in the chopped walnuts.
6. Pour in an appropriate amount of the batter into your waffle maker and spread out the batter to the edges to cover all the holes on your waffle maker.

7. Close your waffle maker and cook for about 3 minutes or according to your waffle maker's settings.

8. After the cooking cycle, use a plastic or silicone utensil to Remove now the chaffle from your waffle maker.

9. Repeat step 6 to 8 until you have cooked all the batter into chaffles.

10. Serve and top with sour cream or heavy cream.

Basic Mozzarella Chaffles

Cooking: 6 Minutes

Servings: 2

Ingredients

- 1 large organic egg, beaten
- ½ cup Mozzarella cheese, shredded finely

Directions

- Preheat now a mini waffle iron and then grease it.
- Place the egg and Mozzarella cheese and stir to combine in a tiny bowl.
- Place half of the mixture into Preheat nowed waffle iron and cook for about 2-minutes or until golden brown.
- Repeat now with the remaining mixture. Serve warm.

Nutrition:

Calories: 5, Net Carb: 0.4g, Fat: 3.7g, Saturated Fat: 1.5g, Carbohydrates: 0.4g, Dietary Fiber: 0g, Sugar: 0.2g, Protein: 5.2g

Easy Corndog Chaffle Recipe

Preparation: 10 minutes

Cooking: 4 minutes

Servings: 5

Ingredients

- 2 eggs
- 1 cup Mexican cheese blend
- 1 tbs almond flour
- 1/2 tsp cornbread extract
- 1/4 tsp salt
- hot dogs with hot dog sticks

Directions

1. Preheat now corndog waffle maker.
2. In a tiny bowl, whip the eggs.
3. Add the remaining ingredients except the hotdogs
4. Spray the corndog waffle maker with non-stick cooking spray.
5. Fill the corndog waffle maker with the batter halfway filled.

6. Place a stick in the hot dog.
7. Place the hot dog in the batter and slightly press down.
8. Spread a tiny amount of better on top of the hot dog, just enough to fill it.
9. Makes about 4 to 5 chaffle corndogs
10. Cook the corndog chaffles for about 4 minutes or until golden brown.
11. When done, they will easily Remove now from the corndog waffle maker with a pair of tongs.
12. Serve with mustard, mayo, or sugar-free ketchup!

Pumpkin Chaffle With Maple Syrup

Preparation: 10 minutes

Cooking: 16 minutes

Servings: 2

Ingredients

- 2 eggs, beaten
- ½ cup Mozzarella cheese, shredded
- 1 teaspn coconut flour
- ¾ teaspn baking powder
- ¾ teaspn pumpkin pie spice
- 2 teaspns pureed pumpkin
- 4 teaspns heavy whipping cream ½ teaspn vanilla
- Pinch salt
- 2 teaspns maple syrup (sugar-free)

Directions

1. Turn your waffle maker on.
2. Mix all the ingredients except maple syrup in a large bowl.

3. Pour half of the batter into your waffle maker.

4. Close and cooking for minutes.

5. Transfer to a plate to cool for 2 minutes.

6. Repeat the steps with the remaining mixture.

7. Drizzle the maple syrup on top of the chaffles before serving.

Nutrition:

34.5g Protein, 0.4g Carbohydrates, 12.9g Fat, 0.1g Fiber, 117mg Cholesterol, 117mg Sodium, 479mg Potassium.

Keto Chaffle Italian Garlic and Herb

Preparation: 5 minutes+

Cooking: 3-5 minutes

Servings: 1

Ingredients

- ½ Cup of Shredded mozzarella cheese
- 1 Egg
- 1 Tbsp. Almond flour
- ¼ tsp. Garlic powder
- ¼ tsp. Italian seasoning
- 1 Tbsp. Heavy whipping cream
- ¼ C. Grated parmesan cheese

Directions

1. Preheat now your mini waffle maker.
2. Mix now the Ingredients for the chaffle in a mixing bowl until completely combined. This mixture will not be liquidy like most waffle batters, it is supposed to have a more solid consistency.

3. Spread half of the mixture evenly into the mini waffle maker, and cook for 3-5 minutes until it is done to your liking.
4. Remove now the first chaffle, and put the second half of the batter into the mini waffle maker.

Nutrition:

6 net carbs per serving

Almonds Chaffle

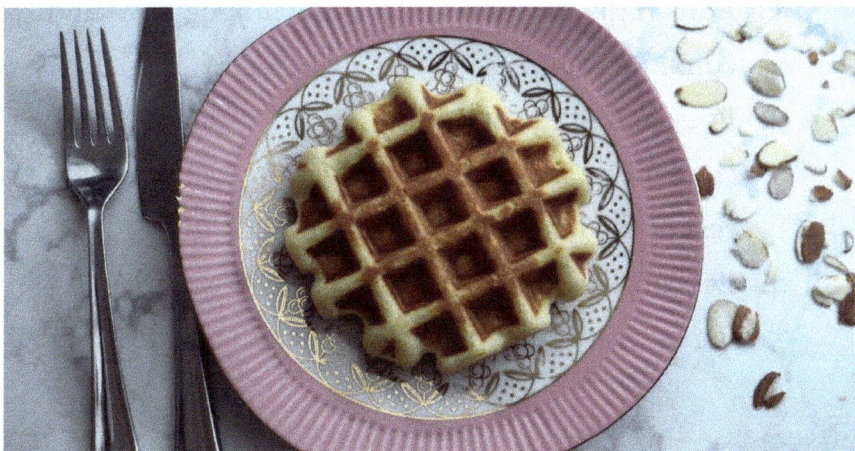

Preparation: 4 minutes

Cooking: 8 minutes

Servings: 2 chaffles

Ingredients

- 1 large egg, beaten
- ½ cup of mozzarella cheese, shredded
- 2 tbsp almond flour
- ¼ tsp baking powder
- 2 tbsp almonds, chopped

Directions

1. Heat up your waffle maker.
2. Add all the ingredients to a tiny mixing bowl and combine well.
3. Pour half of the batter into your waffle maker and cook for 4 minutes until brown. Repeat now with the rest of the batter to make another chaffle.
4. Let cool for 3 minutes to let chaffles get crispy.
5. Serve with keto whipped cream and enjoy!

Maple Syrup & Vanilla Chaffle

Preparation: 10 minutes

Cooking: 12 minutes

Servings: 3

Ingredients

- 1 egg, beaten
- ¼ cup Mozzarella cheese, shredded
- 1 oz. cream cheese
- 1 teaspn vanilla
- 1 tbspn keto maple syrup
- 1 teaspn sweetener
- 1 teaspn baking powder
- 4 tbsps almond flour

Directions

1. Preheat now your waffle maker.
2. Add all the ingredients to a bowl.
3. Mix well.
4. Pour some of the batter into your waffle maker.

5. Cover and cooking for 4 minutes.

6. Transfer chaffle to a plate and let cool for 2 minutes.

7. Repeat the same process with the remaining mixture.

Nutrition:

Calories per servings: 515; Carbohydrates: 2.5g; Protein: 39.2g; Fat: 34.3g; Sugar: 0g; Sodium: 613mg; Fiber:0.9 g

Keto Wonder Bread Chaffle (Coconut and Almond Flour Version)

Preparation: 20 minutes

Servings: 1

Ingredients

- 1 Tbspn Coconut flour
- 1 Tbspn Water
- 1 Tbspn Dukes Mayonnaise
- 1/8 Teaspn Baking Powder
- 1 egg
- Pinch of pink Himalayan salt

Directions

1. Mix all the Ingredients in a tiny bowl. Allow the batter to sit for about a minute to thicken and stir it again.
2. Pour half the batter into your waffle maker and cook for about 2 1/2 to 3 minutes or until golden brown.

Nutrition:

Calories: 123kcal, Carbohydrates: 5.4g, Protein: 4.5g, Fat: 8.6g, Fiber: 1.5g

Celery and Cottage Cheese Chaffle

Preparation: 10 minutes

Cooking: 15 minutes

Servings: 4

Ingredients

- 4 eggs
- 2 cups grated cheddar cheese
- 1 cup fresh celery, chopped
- Salt and pepper to taste
- 2 tbsps chopped almonds
- 2 teaspns baking powder
- 2 tbsps cooking spray to brush your waffle maker ¼ cup cottage cheese for serving

Directions

1. Preheat now your waffle maker.
2. Add the eggs, grated Mozzarella cheese, chopped celery, salt and pepper, chopped almonds and baking powder to a bowl.
3. Mix with a fork.

4. Brush the heated waffle maker with cooking spray and add a few tbsps of the batter.
5. Close the lid and cooking for about 7 minutes depending on your waffle maker.
6. Serve each chaffle with cottage cheese on top.

Nutrition:

Calories 292, Fat 12, Fiber 3, Carbs 7, Protein 16

Vanilla Keto Chaffle

Preparation: 3 min

Cooking: 4 min

Servings: 1

Ingredients

- 1 egg
- 1/2 cup cheddar cheese, shredded
- 1/2 tsp vanilla extract

Directions

1. Switch on your waffle maker according to manufacturer's Directions
2. Crack egg and combine with cheddar cheese in a tiny bowl
3. Add vanilla extract and combine thoroughly.
4. Place half batter on waffle maker and spread evenly.
5. Cook for 4 minutes or until as desired
6. Gently Remove now from waffle maker and set aside for 2 minutes so it cools down and become crispy
7. Repeat for remaining batter

Crispy Sandwich Chaffle

Preparation: 3 min

Cooking: 4 min

Servings: 1

Ingredients

- 1 egg
- 1/2 cup cheddar cheese, shredded
- 1 tbsp coconut flour

Directions:

1. Using a mini waffle maker, Preheat now according to maker's Directions.
2. Combine egg and cheddar cheese in a mixing bowl. Stir thoroughly
3. Add coconut flour for added texture if so desired
4. Place half batter on waffle maker and spread evenly.
5. Cook for 4 minutes or until as desired
6. Gently Remove now from waffle maker and set aside for 2 minutes so it cools down and become crispy
7. Repeat for remaining batter
8. Stuff 2 chaffles with desired sandwich

Yogurt Chaffles

Cooking: 10 Minutes

Servings: 3

Ingredients

- ½ cup shredded mozzarella
- 1 egg
- 2 Tbsp ground almonds
- ½ tsp psyllium husk
- ¼ tsp baking powder
- 1 Tbsp yogurt

Directions

1. Turn on waffle maker to heat and oil it with cooking spray.
2. Whisk eggs in a bowl.
3. Add in remaining ingredients except mozzarella and mix well.
4. Add mozzarella and mix once again. Let it sit for 5 minutes.
5. Add ⅓ cup batter into each waffle mold.

6. Close and cook for 4-5 minutes.

7. Repeat now with remaining batter.

Nutritio :

Carbs: 2 g, Fat: 5 g, Protein: 4 g, Calories: 93

Simple Chaffles Without Maker

Preparation: 6 minutes

Cooking: 5 Minutes

Servings: 2

Ingredients

- 1 tbsp. chia seeds
- 1 egg
- 1/2 cup cheddar cheese
- pinch of salt
- 1 tbsp. avocado oil

Directions

1. Heat your nonstick pan over medium heat
2. In a tiny bowl, mix chia seeds, salt, egg, and cheese together
3. Grease pan with avocado oil.
4. Once the pan is hot, pour 2 tbsps. chaffle batter and cooking for about 1-2 minutes.
5. Flip and cooking for another 1-2 minutes.

6. Once chaffle is brown Remove now from pan.

7. Serve with berries on top and enjoy.

Nutrition:

Calories 100, Fat 7.1, Fiber 2.3, Carbs 5.2, Protein 5.5

Herb Chaffles

Cooking: 12 Minutes

Servings: 4

Ingredients

- 4 tbsps almond flour
- 1 tbspn coconut flour
- 1 teaspn mixed dried herbs
- 1/2 teaspn organic baking powder
- 1/4 teaspn garlic powder
- 1/4 teaspn onion powder
- Salt and ground black pepper, to taste
- 1/4 cup cream cheese, softened
- 3 large organic eggs
- 1/2 cup cheddar cheese, grated
- 1/3 cup of Parmesan cheese, grated

Directions

1. Preheat now a waffle iron and then grease it.
2. In a bowl, mix now the flours, dried herbs, baking powder, seasoning, and mix well.

3. In a separate bowl, put cream cheese and eggs and beat until well combined.
4. Add the flour mixture, cheddar, Parmesan cheese, and Mix well until well combined.
5. Place the desired amount of the mixture into Preheat nowed waffle iron and cook for about 2-3 minutes.
6. Repeat now with the remaining mixture.
7. Serve warm.

Nutrition:

Calories 240, Total Fat 19 g, Saturated Fat 5 g, Cholesterol 176 mg, Sodium 280 mg, Total Carbs 4 g, Fiber 1.6 g, Sugar 0.7 g, Protein 12.3 g

Scallion Chaffles

Cooking: 8 Minutes

Servings: 2

Ingredients

- 1 organic egg, beaten
- 1/2 cup Mozzarella cheese, shredded
- 1 tbspn scallion, chopped
- 1/2 teaspn Italian seasoning

Directions

1. Preheat now a mini waffle iron and then grease it.
2. In a bowl, place all ingredients and with a fork, Mix well until well combined.
3. Place half of the mixture into Preheat nowed waffle iron and cook for about 4 minutes or until golden brown.
4. Repeat now with the remaining mixture.
5. Serve warm.

Nutrition:

Carb:0.7g, Fat: 3.8g, Saturated Fat: 1.5 g, Carbohydrates:0.8g, Dietary Fiber: 0 g, Sugar: 0.3g, Protein: 4.8g

Basic Keto Chaffle

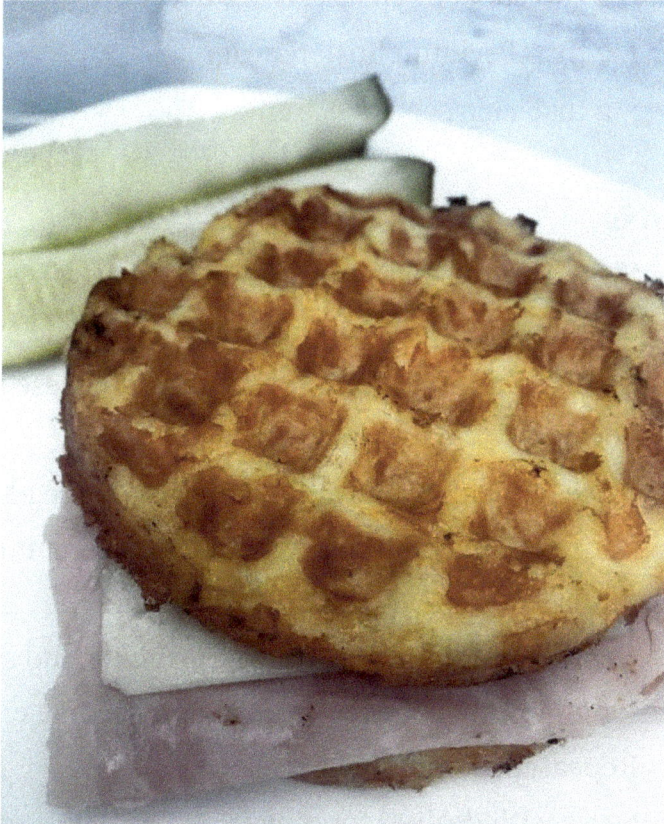

Preparation: 3 min

Cooking: 4 min

Servings: 1

Ingredients

- 1 egg
- 1/2 cup cheddar cheese, shredded
- 1/2 tbsp Psyllium husk powder
- 1/2 tbsp chia seeds

Directions:

1. Switch on your waffle maker according to manufacturer's Directions
2. Crack egg and combine with cheddar cheese in a tiny bowl
3. Place half batter on waffle maker and spread evenly.
4. Sprinkle Chia on top, cover and cook for 4 minutes or until as desired
5. Gently Remove now from waffle maker and set aside for 2 minutes so it cools down and become crispy
6. Repeat for remaining batter
7. Serve with desired toppings

Sandwich Chaffle

Preparation: 3 min

Cooking: 4 min

Servings: 1

Ingredients

- 1 egg
- 1/2 cup cheddar cheese, shredded
- 1 tbsp almond flour (optional)

Directions:

1. Using a mini waffle maker, Preheat now according to maker's Directions.
2. Combine egg and cheddar cheese in a mixing bowl. Stir thoroughly
3. Add Almond flour for added texture if so desired; mix well
4. Place half batter on waffle maker and spread evenly.
5. Cook for 4 minutes or until as desired
6. Gently Remove now from waffle maker and set aside for 2 minutes so it cools down and become crispy
7. Repeat for remaining batter

8. Stuff 2 chaffles with desired garnishing to make a sandwich

Nutrition:

170 calories, 2g net carbs, 14g fat, 10g protein

Flaky Delight Chaffle

Preparation: 3 min

Cooking: 4 min

Servings: 1

Ingredients

- 1 egg
- 1/2 cup cheddar cheese, shredded
- 1/2 cup coconut flakes

Directions

1. Switch on your waffle maker according to manufacturer's Directions
2. Crack egg and combine with cheddar cheese in a tiny bowl
3. Place half batter on waffle maker and spread evenly.
4. Sprinkle coconut flakes and Cook for 4 minutes or until as desired
5. Gently Remove now from waffle maker and set aside for 2 minutes so it cools down and become crispy
6. Repeat for remaining batter

7. Serve with desired toppings

Nutrition:

291 calories, 1g net carbs, 23g fat, 20g protein

Keto Minty Base Chaffle

Preparation: 3 min

Cooking: 4 min

Servings: 1

Ingredients

- 1 egg
- 1/2 cup cheddar cheese, shredded
- 1 tbsp mint extract (low carb)

Directions

1. Using a mini waffle maker, Preheat now according to maker's Directions.
2. Combine egg and cheddar cheese in a mixing bowl. Stir thoroughly
3. Add mint extract and place half batter on waffle maker; spread evenly.
4. Cook for 4 minutes or until as desired
5. Gently Remove now from waffle maker and set aside for 2 minutes so it cools down and become crispy
6. Repeat for remaining batter

7. Garnish with desired toppings

Nutrition:

170 calories, 2g net carbs, 14g fat, 10g protein

Chocolate Melt now Chaffles

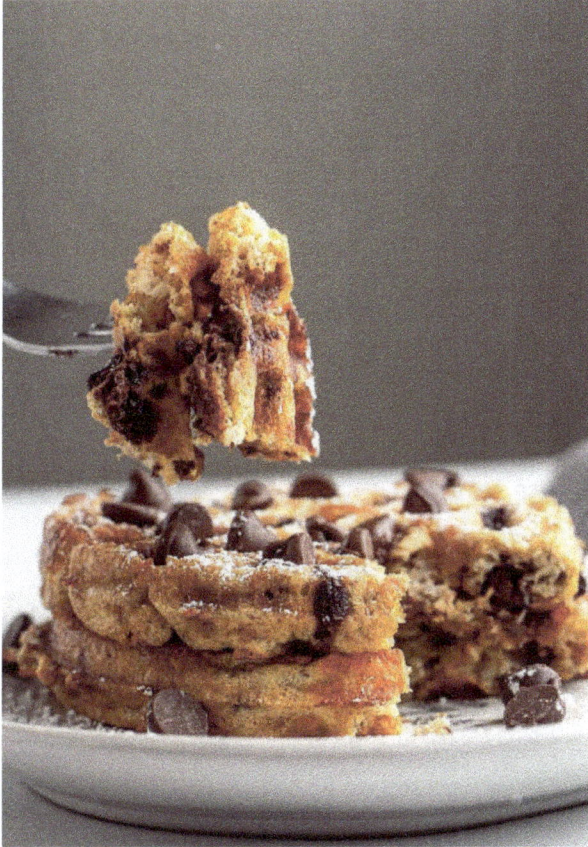

Preparation: 9 minutes

Cooking: 36 Minutes

Servings: 2

Ingredients

For the chaffles:

- 2 eggs, beaten
- ¼ cup finely grated Gruyere cheese
- 2 tbsp heavy cream
- 1 tbsp coconut flour
- 2 tbsp cream cheese, softened
- 3 tbsp unsweetened cocoa powder
- 2 tsp vanilla extract
- A pinch of salt

For the chocolate sauce:

- 1/3 cup of + 1 tbsp heavy cream
- 1 ½ oz unsweetened baking chocolate, chopped
- 1 ½ tsp sugar-free maple syrup
- 1 ½ tsp vanilla extract

Directions

For the chaffles:

1. Preheat now the waffle iron.
2. In a bowl, mix all the ingredients for the chaffles.
3. Open the iron and add a quarter of the mixture. Close and cook until crispy, 7 minutes.
4. Transfer the chaffle to a plate and make 3 more with the remaining batter.

<u>For the chocolate sauce:</u>

1. Pour the heavy cream into saucepan and simmer over low heat, 3 minutes.
2. Turn the heat off and add the chocolate. Allow Melt nowing for a few minutes and stir until fully Melt nowed, 5 minutes.
3. Mix in the maple syrup and vanilla extract.
4. Assemble the chaffles in layers with the chocolate sauce sandwiched between each layer.
5. Slice and serve immediately.

Nutrition:

Calories 338, Total Fat 3.8 g, Saturated Fat 0.7 g, Cholesterol 22 mg, Total Carbs 8.3 g, Fiber 2.4 g, Sugar 1.2 g, Sodium 620 mg, Potassium 271 mg, Protein 15.4g

Zucchini Chaffles

Cooking: 18 Minutes

Servings: 4

Ingredients

- 2 large zucchinis, grated and squeezed
- 2 large organic eggs
- 2/3 cup Cheddar cheese, shredded
- 2 tbsps coconut flour
- 1/2 teaspn garlic powder
- 1/2 teaspn red pepper flakes, crushed
- Salt, to taste

Directions

1. Preheat now a waffle iron and then grease it.
2. Place all ingredients and Mix well until well combined in a bowl.
3. Place 1/4 of the mixture into Preheat nowed waffle iron and cook for about 4-41/z minutes or until golden brown.
4. Repeat now with the remaining mixture.

72

5. Serve warm.

Nutrition:

Calories: 1 59, Net Carb: 4.3 g, Fat: 10g, Saturated Fat: 5.8g, Carbohydrates: 8g, Dietary Fiber: 3.7g, Sugar: 2g, Protein: 10.1g

Chaffle Bread Sticks

Preparation: 10 minutes

Cooking: 13 minutes

Servings: 2 medium chaffles

Ingredients

For Chaffles:

- 2 tbsps almond flour
- 1/2 teaspn dried oregano
- 1/2 teaspn garlic powder
- 1/2 teaspn salt
- 1/2 cup / 60 grams grated mozzarella cheese
- 1 egg, at room temperature

For Topping:

- 1/4 cup / 30 grams grated mozzarella cheese
- 1/2 teaspn garlic powder
- 2 tbsps coconut butter, unsalted, softened

Directions

1. Take a non-stick waffle iron, plug it in, select the medium or medium-high heat setting and let it Preheat now until ready to use; it could also be indicated with an indicator light changing its color.

2. Meanwhile, prepare the batter and for this, take a large bowl, crack the egg in it, add flour, oregano, garlic powder, salt, and mozzarella cheese and mix with an electric mixer until incorporated.

3. Use a spoon to pour half of the prepared batter into the heated waffle iron in a spiral direction, starting from the edges, then shut the lid and cook for 5 minutes or more until solid and nicely browned; the cooked waffle will look like a cake.

4. When done, transfer chaffles to a plate with a silicone spatula and Repeat now with the remaining batter.

5. Meanwhile, prepare the topping and for this, take a tiny bowl, add garlic and butter in it and stir well until combined.

6. Let chaffles stand until crispy, then arrange them on a heatproof tray, and drizzle the topping on top.

7. Preheat now the grill over medium-high heat, and when hot, place the tray containing chaffle sticks and grill for 3 minutes until cheese has Melt nowed.

8. Serve straight away.

Pumpkin & Pecan Chaffle

Preparation: 10 minutes

Cooking: 10 Minutes

Servings: 2

Ingredients

- 1 egg, beaten
- ½ cup mozzarella cheese, grated
- ½ teaspn pumpkin spice
- 1 tbspn pureed pumpkin
- 2 tbsps almond flour
- 1 teaspn sweetener
- 2 tbsps pecans, chopped

Directions

1. Turn on your waffle maker.
2. Beat the egg in a bowl.
3. Stir in the rest of the ingredients.
4. Pour half of the mixture into the device.
5. Seal the lid.
6. Cook for 5 minutes.

7. Remove now the chaffle carefully.

8. Repeat the steps to make the second chaffle.

Nutrition:

Calories 604, Total Fat 30.6 g, Saturated Fat 13.1 g, Cholesterol 131 mg, Total Carbs 1.4g, Fiber 0.2 g, Sugar 20.3 g, Sodium 834 mg, Potassium 512 mg, Protein 54.6 g

Gingerbread Chaffle

Cooking: 5 Minutes

Servings: 2

Ingredients

- ½ cup mozzarella cheese grated
- 1 medium egg
- ½ tsp baking powder
- 1 tsp erythritol powdered
- ½ tsp ground ginger
- ¼ tsp ground nutmeg
- ½ tsp ground cinnamon
- ⅛ tsp ground cloves
- 2 Tbsp almond flour
- 1 cup heavy whipped cream
- ¼ cup keto-friendly maple syrup

Directions

1. Turn on waffle maker to heat and oil it with cooking spray.
2. Beat egg in a bowl.

3. Add flour, mozzarella, spices, baking powder, and erythritol. Mix well.
4. Spoon one half of the batter into waffle maker and spread out evenly.
5. Close and cook for minutes.
6. Remove now cooked chaffle and Repeat now with remaining batter.
7. Serve with whipped cream and maple syrup.

Nutrition:

Carbs: 5 g, Fat: 15 g, Protein: 12 g, Calories: 103

Almond Flour Chaffles

Cooking: 20 Minutes

Servings: 2

Ingredients

- 1 large egg
- 1 Tbsp blanched almond flour
- ¼ tsp baking powder
- ½ cup shredded mozzarella cheese

Directions

1. Whisk egg, almond flour, and baking powder together.
2. Stir in mozzarella and set batter aside.
3. Turn on waffle maker to heat and oil it with cooking spray.
4. Pour half of the batter onto waffle maker and spread it evenly with a spoon.
5. Cook for 3 min, or until it reaches desired doneness.
6. Transfer to a plate and Repeat now with remaining batter.

7. Let chaffles cool for 2-3 minutes to crisp up.

Nutrition:

Carbs: 2 g, Fat: 13 g, Protein: 10 g, Calories: 131

Cinnamon Garlic Chaffles

Preparation: 5 minutes

Cooking: 10 minutes

Servings: 2

Ingredients

- Egg: 1
- Mozzarella cheese: ½ cup (shredded)
- Garlic: ½ tbsp. ground
- Ground cinnamon: ½ tsp.
- Erythritol: 1 tsp. powdered
- Ground nutmeg: ¼ tsp.
- Almond flour: 2 tbsp.
- Baking powder: ½ tsp.

Directions

1. Mix all the ingredients well together
2. Pour a layer on a Preheat nowed waffle iron
3. Cooking the chaffle for around 5 minutes
4. Make as many chaffles as your mixture and waffle maker allow

5. Serve with your favorite topping

Nutrition:

Calories: 288; Total Fat: 24g; Carbs: 7g; Net Carbs: 4g; Fiber: 3g; Protein: 14g

Coconut Flour Waffle

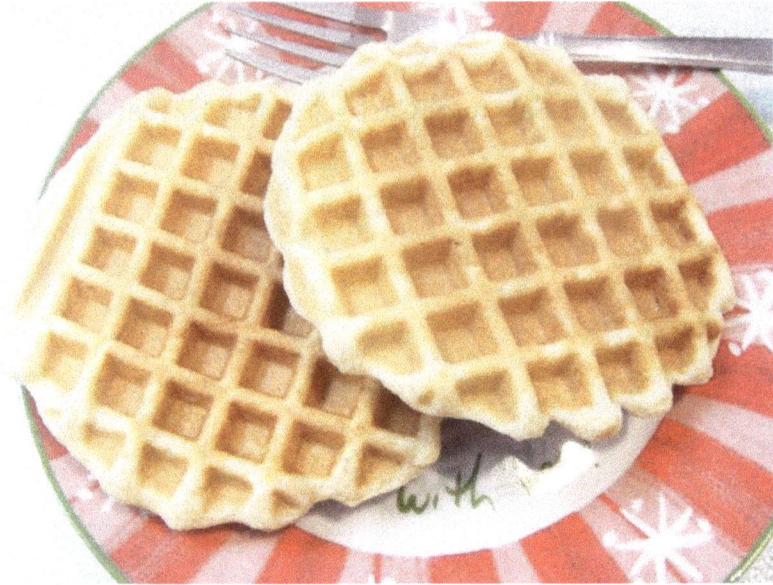

Preparation: 5 minutes

Cooking: 5 minutes

Servings: 4

Ingredients

- 8 eggs
- 1/2 cup of butter or coconut oil (Melt nowed)
- 1 tsp. of vanilla extract
- 1/2 tsp. salt

84

- 1/2 cup of coconut flour

Directions

1. Pre heat the mini waffle maker,
2. Whisk the eggs in a bowl,
3. You add the Melt nowed butter or coconut oil, cinnamon, vanilla and salt, mix properly, and add the Coconut flour.
4. Ensure the batter is thick,
5. Add the mixture into the mini waffle maker and cook until it has a light brown appearance.
6. Serve with butter or maple syrup.

Nutrition:

Net Carbs: 6.8g; Calories: 357; Total Fat: 28.9g; Saturated Fat: 13.2g; Protein: 15.2g; Carbs: 8.9g; Fiber: 2.1g; Sugar: 3.9g

Garlic powder & Oregano Chaffles

Cooking: 10 Minutes

Servings: 2

Ingredients

- 1/2 cup Mozzarella cheese, grated
- 1 medium organic egg, beaten
- 2 tbsps almond flour
- 1/2 teaspn dried oregano, crushed
- 1/2 teaspn garlic powder
- Salt, to taste

Directions

1. Preheat now a mini waffle iron and then grease it.
2. In a bowl, place all ingredients and Mix well until well combined.
3. Place half of the mixture into Preheat nowed waffle iron and cook for about 4-5 minutes or until golden brown.
4. Repeat now with the remaining mixture.
5. Serve warm.

Nutrition:

Calories: 100, Net Carb: 1.4g, Fat: 7.2 g, Saturated Fat: 1.7g, Carbohydrates: 2.4g, Sugar: 0, Protein:4.9g

Cream Cheese Waffle

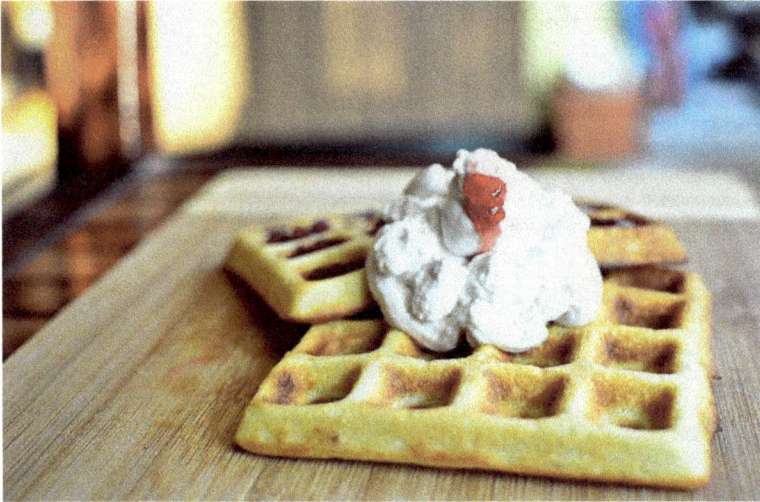

Preparation: 10 minutes

Cooking: 5 minutes

Servings: 4

Ingredients

- 2 cups of flour
- 1 tsp. baking powder
- 1/8 tsp. salt
- 2 tsp. light brown sugar
- 4-ounce of 1/3 Less Fat Cream Cheese

- 2 eggs
- 1/2 cups of milk
- 2 tbsps canola oil
- 1/2 tbspn pure vanilla extract
- 4 tbsps honey

Directions

1. First step is to Preheat now the mini waffle maker.
2. You mix now the flour, baking powder, salt and light brown sugar; mix thoroughly to ensure uniformity.
3. Add the cream cheese and egg yolks; Mix well until smooth.
4. Then you Add milk, oil and vanilla; mix properly.
5. Add flour mixture to cream cheese mixture and stir until moist. Set
6. The next step is to Place egg whites in a bowl and beat until it forms a stiff peak.
7. Using a spatula, fold the egg whites gently into the waffle-batter; fold just until thoroughly combined.
8. Pour 1/3-cup of the batter onto the Preheat nowed mini waffle iron.
9. Allow to cooking for about 2 to 3 min, or until it has a light brown appearance

10. Next step is to the Whipped Cream. Pour the heavy cream into a large mixing bowl and beat on until it becomes thick.
11. Add honey and continue to beat until soft peaks form. When ready,
12. Serve waffles topped with Honey Whipped Cream and fresh berries (if you prefer).

Nutrition:

Net Carbs: 3.5g: 202.5; Total Fat: 24.2g; Saturated Fat: 6g; Protein: 22.7g; Carbs: 4g; Fiber: 0.5g; Sugar: 1.1g

Sugar Free Sprinkles Chaffle

Preparation: 5 minutes

Cooking: 8 minutes

Servings: 2 chaffles

Ingredients

- 1 egg
- ½ cup shredded mozzarella cheese
- 1 tbsp almond flour
- 1 tbsp heavy whipping cream
- ½ tsp vanilla extract
- 1 tbsp sugar free sprinkles
- 2 tsp sweetener

Directions

1. Heat up the mini waffle maker.
2. Add all the ingredients to a tiny mixing bowl and combine well.

3. Pour half of the batter into your waffle maker and cook for 4 minutes. Repeat now with the rest of the batter to make another chaffle.
4. Let cool for 3 minutes to let chaffles get crispy.
5. Top the chaffle with some sugar free whipped cream and a few sugar free sprinkles.
6. Serve and enjoy!

Mayonnaise Chaffle

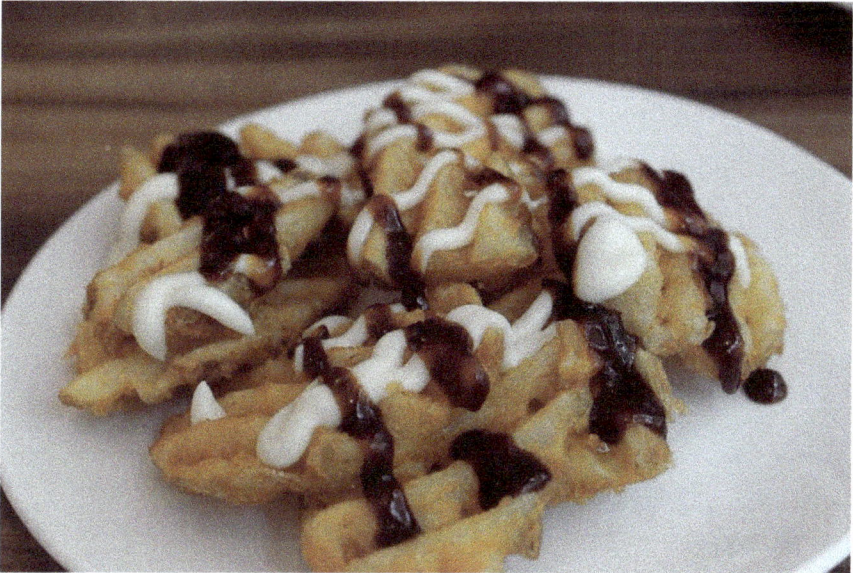

Preparation: 5 minutes

Cooking: 10 Minutes

Servings: 3

Ingredients

- 1 large organic egg, beaten1 tbspn mayonnaise
- 2 tbsps almond flour
- 1/8 teaspn organic baking powder

- 1 teaspn water2–4 drops liquid stevia

Directions

1. Preheat now a mini waffle iron and then grease it.
2. In a bowl, put all ingredients and Mix well until well combined with a fork. Place half of the mixture into Preheat nowed waffle iron and cooking for about 4–5 minutes.
3. Repeat now with the remaining mixture.
4. Serve warm.

Nutrition:

Calories 208, Fat 7, Carbs 22, Protein 19

Light & Crispy Bacon Cheddar Chaffles Recipe

Preparation: 5 minutes

Cooking: 5 minutes

Servings: 4

Ingredients

- 2 eggs
- 1 cup cheddar
- ½ Coconut/almond flour
- 1/2 teaspn baking powder
- Bacon
- Shredded parmesan cheese on top and bottom.

Directions

1. Heat up the waffle iron on medium.
2. Mix eggs, cheddar cheese in a tiny bowl.
3. Whisk egg thoroughly
4. Mix flour, baking powder, salt together in a large bowl

5. Gently whisk the egg mixture into the dry ingredients.
6. Whisk thoroughly until smooth
7. Add the bacon into the mixture and mix thoroughly
8. Lightly grease the waffle iron
9. Spoon the batter into your waffle maker
10. Bake till crispy and golden brown.
11. Repeat baking procedure till batter is finished.
12. Serve warm.

Nutrition:

Calories 129, Fat 11.7, Fiber 2.7, Carbs 5.8, Protein 2.2

Garlic Powdered Chaffles

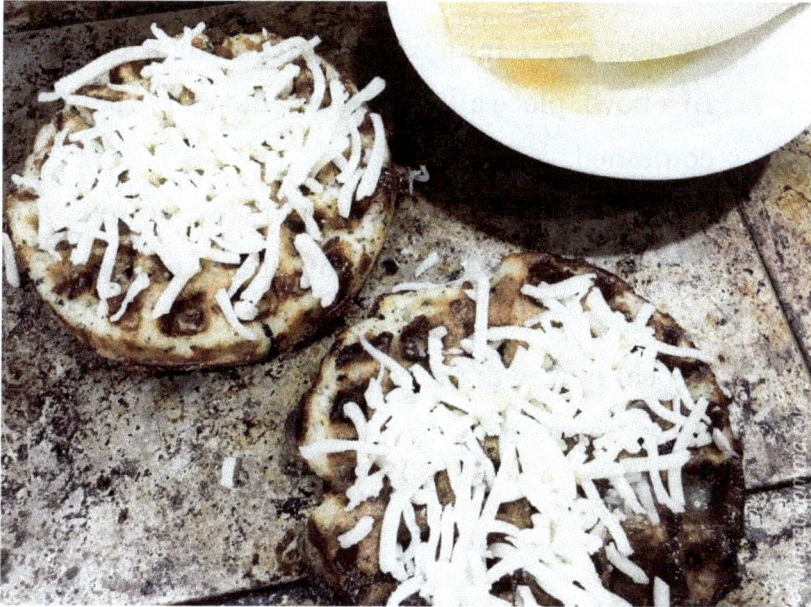

Preparation: 6 minutes

Cooking: 8 Minutes

Servings: 2

Ingredients

- 1 organic egg, beaten
- ½ cup Monterrey Jack cheese, shredded
- 1 teaspn coconut flour

- Pinch of garlic powder

Directions:

1. Preheat now a mini waffle iron and then grease it.
2. In a bowl, place all the ingredients and beat until well combined.
3. Place half of the mixture into Preheat nowed waffle iron and cook for about 4 minutes or until golden brown.
4. Repeat now with the remaining mixture.
5. Serve warm.

Nutrition:

Calories 34, Fat 1.3, Fiber 3.6, Carbs 4.7, Protein 3.6

Chaffle with Garlic

Preparation: 5 minutes

Cooking: 8 minutes

Servings: 2 chaffles

Ingredients

- 1 egg, beaten
- ½ cup shredded mozzarella cheese
- ¼ tsp garlic powder

Directions

1. Heat up your waffle maker.
2. Add egg, shredded mozzarella cheese and garlic powder to a tiny mixing bowl and combine well.
3. Pour half of the batter into your waffle maker and cook for 4 minutes. Repeat now with the rest of the batter to make another chaffle.
4. Let cool for 3 minutes to let chaffles get crispy.
5. Serve and enjoy!

Parsley Chaffle

Preparation: 5 minutes

Cooking: 8 minutes

Servings: 2 chaffles

Ingredients

- 1 egg, beaten
- ½ cup shredded mozzarella cheese
- ½ tbsp fresh parsley, finely chopped

Directions

1. Heat up your waffle maker.
2. Add egg, shredded mozzarella cheese and parsley to a tiny mixing bowl and combine well.
3. Pour half of the batter into your waffle maker and cook for 4 minutes until brown. Repeat now with the rest of the batter to make another chaffle.
4. Serve and enjoy!

Fresh Basil Chaffle

Preparation: 5 minutes

Cooking: 8 minutes

Servings: 2 chaffles

Ingredients

- 1 egg, beaten
- ½ cup shredded cheddar cheese
- ½ tbsp fresh basil, finely chopped

Directions

1. Heat up your waffle maker.
2. Add egg, shredded cheddar cheese, and basil to a tiny mixing bowl and combine well.
3. Pour half of the batter into your waffle maker and cook for 4 minutes until brown. Repeat now with the rest of the batter to make another chaffle.
4. Serve with a slice of tomato and keto mayonnaise and enjoy!

Provolone Cheese Chaffle

Preparation: 5 minutes

Cooking: 8 minutes

Servings: 2 chaffles

Ingredients

- 1 egg, beaten
- ½ cup shredded Provolone cheese

Directions

1. Heat up your waffle maker.
2. Add egg and shredded cheese to a tiny mixing bowl and combine well.
3. Pour half of the batter into your waffle maker and cook for 4 minutes until brown. Repeat now with the rest of the batter to make another chaffle.
4. Let cool for 3 minutes to let chaffles get crispy.
5. Serve and enjoy!

Corn Bread Chaffle

Preparation: 10 minutes

Cooking: 20 minutes

Servings: 4 medium chaffles

Ingredients

- 3 cups / 290 grams ground almonds, blanched
- 2 teaspns baking soda
- 8 tbsps hemp seeds
- 1 teaspn baking powder
- 1 teaspn of sea salt
- 4 tbsps avocado oil
- 8 tbsps coconut milk, unsweetened
- 4 eggs, at room temperature

Directions

1. Take a non-stick waffle iron, plug it in, select the medium or medium-high heat setting and let it Preheat now until ready to use; it could also be indicated with an indicator light changing its color.

2. Meanwhile, prepare the batter and for this, take a large bowl, add almonds and seeds in it and then stir in salt, baking powder, and soda until combined.

3. Take a separate bowl, crack eggs in it, add oil, pour in milk, stir with a hand whisk until frothy, and then stir this mixture with a spoon into the almond mixture until incorporated.

4. Use a spoon to pour one-fourth of the prepared batter into the heated waffle iron in a spiral direction, starting from the edges, then shut the lid and cook for 5 minutes or more until solid and nicely browned; the cooked waffle will look like a cake.

5. When done, transfer chaffles to a plate with a silicone spatula and Repeat now with the remaining batter.

6. Let chaffles stand for some time until crispy and serve straight away.

Cheesy Chaffle

Preparation: 5 minutes

Cooking: 8 minutes

Servings: 2 chaffles

Ingredients

- 1 large egg, beaten
- ½ cup shredded Cheddar cheese
- ½ tsp ground flaxseed
- ¼ tsp baking powder
- 2 tbsp shredded Parmesan cheese

Directions

1. Heat up the mini waffle maker.
2. Add all the ingredients except Parmesan cheese to a tiny mixing bowl and stir until well combined.
3. Pour half of the Parmesan cheese in the Preheat nowed waffle maker.
4. Pour half of the batter into your waffle maker, top with the remaining Parmesan cheese and cook for 4

minutes until brown. Repeat now with the remaining batter/cheese to prepare another chaffle.

5. Let cool for 3 minutes to let chaffles get crispy.
6. Serve and enjoy!

Parmesan Cheese Chaffle

Preparation: 5 minutes

Cooking: 8 minutes

Servings: 2 chaffles

Ingredients

- 1 large egg, beaten
- ½ cup Parmesan cheese, finely grated
- A pinch of salt and pepper

Directions

1. Heat up your waffle maker.
2. Add all the ingredients to a tiny mixing bowl and combine well.
3. Pour half of the batter into your waffle maker and cook for 4 minutes until golden brown. Repeat now with the rest of the batter to make another chaffle.
4. Let cool for 3 minutes to let chaffles get crispy.
5. Serve and enjoy!

Swiss Cheese Chaffle

Preparation: 5 minutes

Cooking: 8 minutes

Servings: 2 chaffles

Ingredients

- 1 large egg, beaten
- ½ cup of Swiss cheese, shredded
- 1 tbsp almond flour

Directions

1. Heat up your waffle maker.
2. Add the cheese, almond flour, and egg to a tiny mixing bowl and combine well.
3. Pour half of the batter into your waffle maker and cook for 4 minutes until golden brown. Repeat now with the rest of the batter to make another chaffle.
4. Let cool for 3 minutes to let chaffles get crispy.
5. Serve and enjoy!

Bread Chaffle

Preparation: 4 minutes

Cooking: 8 minutes

Servings: 2 chaffles

Ingredients

- 1 egg
- 2 tbsp almond flour
- 1 tbsp mayonnaise
- ¼ tsp baking powder
- 1 tsp water

Directions

1. Heat up your waffle maker.
2. In a tiny bowl, whisk the egg until beaten.
3. Mix almond flour, mayonnaise, baking powder, and water in a mixing bowl.
4. Combine egg and flour mixture.

5. Pour half of the batter into your waffle maker and cook for 4 minutes. Repeat now with the rest of the batter to make another chaffle.
6. Serve and enjoy!

Sweet Chaffle

Preparation: 5 minutes

Cooking: 8 minutes

Servings: 2 chaffles

Ingredients

- 1 egg, beaten
- ½ cup mozzarella cheese, shredded
- 1 tbsp cocoa powder, unsweetened
- 2 tbsp almond flour

Directions

1. Heat up your waffle maker.
2. Add all the ingredients to a tiny mixing bowl and stir until well combined.
3. Pour half of the batter into your waffle maker and cook for 4 minutes until golden brown. Repeat now with the rest of the batter to make another chaffle.
4. Serve with strawberries and keto whipped cream and enjoy!

Almond Butter Chaffle

Preparation: 5 minutes

Cooking: 8 minutes

Servings: 2 chaffles

Ingredients

- 1 large egg, beaten
- ½ cup of mozzarella cheese, shredded
- 2 tbsp almond flour
- ¼ tsp baking powder
- 2 tbsp almond butter for topping

Directions

1. Heat up your waffle maker.
2. Add all the ingredients to a tiny mixing bowl and stir until well combined.
3. Pour half of the batter into your waffle maker and cook for 4 minutes. Repeat now with the rest of the batter to make another chaffle.
4. Let cool for 3 minutes to let chaffles get crispy.
5. Spread the chaffles with almond butter.
6. Serve and enjoy!

www.ingramcontent.com/pod-product-compliance
Lightning Source LLC
Chambersburg PA
CBHW050748030426
42336CB00012B/1707